Introduction

Choosing Flower Essences: An Assessment Guide is intended as an evaluation and teaching tool, to be used either by professional practitioners in a counseling format or for independent reflection. This guide lists three or four leading questions pertaining to behaviors and feelings correlated to each flower essence. Beside each question is the opportunity to designate whether these behaviors and feelings are nearly **Always** present, occur **Sometimes,** or are almost **Never** present (indicated by the letters **A, S,** and **N** over the check-off boxes.) The following is a summary of ways in which practitioners may choose to use the Assessment Guide.

Client Intake and Assessment

The Assessment Guide can be used to survey the range of emotions, feelings and behaviors which are germane to flower essence therapy. Once the client has completed this guide, the practitioner can then evaluate the information. Each question is framed so that a positive answer of **Always (A)** indicates a strong possibility for that essence. A response of **Sometimes (S)** indicates an essence or issue that may be in need of further consideration during the counseling session. The Assessment Guide is not intended to provide an exact "scoring" card or mathematical formula for automatically assigning a particular flower essence. If this were so it would deny the client relationship within the full context of the practitioner's healing art. The Guide is intended to provide a time of earnest reflection and inner consideration for the client, which should then be explored within a more active counseling matrix.

Counseling Tool For the Practitioner

In some cases, it may be more appropriate for the counselor or practitioner to use the guide as a reference tool for interviewing the client, rather than have the client answer the questions directly. The Assessment Guide can be an invaluable counseling aid as the practitioner hones in on the specific areas of dysfunction or disharmony for each client. The leading questions listed for each essence will often be trigger points for further discussion about the feelings and situations which are unique to the client. The Assessment Guide can promote a dynamic counseling process leading to selection of appropriate flower essences.

In addition to the data and observations which can be gleaned by using the Assessment Guide, it is recommended that the practitioner consult the *Flower Essence Repertory*, which contains comprehensive descriptions of each essence, as well as an extensive listing of issues and situations associated with flower essence therapy.

For Self-Reflection and Inner Awareness

The Assessment Guide can also be used for personal growth and reflection. By taking the time to honestly consider the questions related to each flower, many insights about one's behavior and feelings can come to the surface.

Those questions which evoke strong feelings can be used as catalysts for journal writing, imagery, affirmations, or other ways in which one explores the meaning and healing potential associated with each flower essence. Following the selection and use of the appropriate flower essences, one can return to these questions at a later time to evaluate one's progress. Frequently, a change in behavior or feelings will be noted, or the guide may reveal new areas needing attention and inner work.

Even though the Assessment Guide can be used for personal exploration, it is still highly recommended that you seek out the advice or insights of family, friends, or co-workers who know you. Ultimately all healing involves a balance between two primary polarities — that of self-responsibility and awareness, and that of social relatedness and reflection. By allowing ourselves to receive help or counsel from others, we are often able to see more deeply into our true nature, and take humble and wise account of our dysfunctional feelings or moral shortcomings.

Directions:

Take a quiet moment to read each of the questions pertaining to each flower. Try to be as honest and spontaneous as possible in choosing your answers. Pause for a moment to consider each question, but do not over-analyze your responses.

Mark "**A**" if the behavior or feeling is always or nearly always present for you.

Mark "**S**" if the behavior or feeling is only sometimes or infrequently present.

Mark "**N**" if you believe that this behavior or feelings is never, or hardly ever present.

You may also wish to mark or underline key words, phrases, or entire questions or essences which evoke an especially strong recognition or emotional response.

Evaluation and Essence Selection:

Please be aware that there is no scoring system associated with this guide. After completing the survey, you should note those essences which contained a response of **"A"** (Always) to one or more of the listed questions. If "A" is marked for all three or four questions in each category, there is a strong likelihood that this flower essence would be beneficial. A particular flower essence may also be indicated if there are two or more **"S"** (Sometimes), or a combination of **"A"** and **"S."** You should also take extra consideration of essences where you have marked key words, phrases, or entire sets of questions as being especially evocative.

Most persons will discover that many questions will show strong responses, indicating far more essences than can be effectively combined in one formula. Further counseling and exploration will be necessary before appropriate selections can be determined. Some important considerations in making a selection include: priorities in development, especially a sense of one's "next step" of progress; the grouping of possible remedies according to key themes such as anger, fear, or depression; the harmonious and effective combination of essences so that there is an energetic wholeness in the formula; and the readiness and willingness of the person to recognize and address the issues represented by the essences.

It is especially recommended that the *Flower Essence Repertory* be consulted for a fuller discussion of counseling and selection principles, as well as more complete descriptions of the flower essences contained in this guide.

Summary

Choosing Flower Essences is meant to be a tool for healing and self-discovery. The Assessment Guide is not meant to replace other methods of professional diagnosis for medical or psychiatric conditions, nor is it meant as a substitute for human-based counseling and other healing relationships. This guide contains profound, leading questions that convey deeper insight about each essence and its possible benefit. However you choose to use this resource, we hope that it may be a positive aid for you in learning the language of the flowers and in experiencing the incredible benefits of flower essence therapy.

A	S	N	## Agrimony
☐	☐	☐	Does it seem that you are wearing a social mask, appearing carefree and cheerful to others, when deep inside you feel quite tormented?
☐	☐	☐	Were you taught to deny your real feelings, to keep a "stiff upper lip," or maintain a veneer of social politeness?
☐	☐	☐	Do you often rely on alcohol or other drugs to keep back any unpleasant or troubling emotions, or to help you to feel at ease?

Aloe Vera

☐	☐	☐	Do you tend to neglect basic emotional or physical needs in order to accomplish goals or projects?
☐	☐	☐	Are you currently in a state of "burn-out" due to a physical, emotional, or otherwise challenging situation?
☐	☐	☐	Would you characterize yourself as a typically "fiery" person with a great deal of enthusiasm and personal ambition?

Alpine Lily

☐	☐	☐	Is it hard for you to relate to the feminine aspect in yourself or others in an earthy or physical way?
☐	☐	☐	**For men:** Do you tend to put women "on a pedestal," or think of them as being more spiritual than physical?
☐	☐	☐	**For women:** Are you currently experiencing congestion or other disturbances in your reproductive system?
☐	☐	☐	**For women:** Is it hard for you to have a positive experience of basic female biological functions such as menstruation, pregnancy, nursing or sexuality?

Angel's Trumpet

☐	☐	☐	Are you going through an intense inner experience, which feels as though some part of you is dying or encountering very deep change?
☐	☐	☐	Do you have a terminal illness which fills you with great fear, because it's hard to think about dying?
☐	☐	☐	Is it difficult for you to surrender or to submit yourself to any process which requires spiritual faith or trust?

A	S	N	

Angelica

☐ ☐ ☐ Do you tend to see others, and the world in general, in purely physical or material terms?

☐ ☐ ☐ Are you going through an experience which requires spiritual protection and guidance?

☐ ☐ ☐ Do you often feel a deep sense of loneliness, as though you are isolated or separated from a spiritual source?

Arnica

☐ ☐ ☐ Have you suffered a major trauma such as an accident or surgery from which you feel you never fully recovered?

☐ ☐ ☐ Are you currently experiencing shock or numbness due to trauma of any kind?

☐ ☐ ☐ Do you feel that you do not fully inhabit some part of your body, or that it is generally difficult for your body to heal from wounds or other injuries?

Aspen

☐ ☐ ☐ Do you often find yourself anxious or fearful, or experience vaguely troubling nightmares, yet are at a loss to understand what is causing or prompting these feelings?

☐ ☐ ☐ Do you seem to have pronounced psychic sensitivity, easily registering impressions from unseen or unknown sources?

☐ ☐ ☐ Do you need to bring more spiritual strength and confidence to your daily life, transforming fear and anxiety to more wakeful perception and inner knowing?

Baby Blue Eyes

☐ ☐ ☐ Is it hard for you to let down your guard around others, or to trust they can help you?

☐ ☐ ☐ Did your early childhood experience include abandonment by your father, or the absence of a loving and supportive father?

☐ ☐ ☐ Do you often have a rather cynical or skeptical attitude toward life, or feel that you must "go it alone"?

Basil

☐ ☐ ☐ Do your values regarding sexuality and spirituality feel in conflict with one another, as though both cannot really exist at the same time?

☐ ☐ ☐ Does your sexuality have a clandestine or secretive aspect to it, such as a hidden love affair?

☐ ☐ ☐ Do you participate in shame-based sexual conduct, or in sexual activities which seem demeaning or dehumanizing?

A	S	N	### Beech

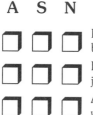

□ □ □ Do you set high standards for others, making it almost impossible for them to live up to your ideals?

□ □ □ Does it seem that you are frequently in a position of criticizing or judging the behavior or performance of others?

□ □ □ Are you hypersensitive to the physical and social environment around you, needing to be surrounded by a "bubble" of perfection?

Black Cohosh

□ □ □ In looking at your family history do you see a pattern of violence or abuse?

□ □ □ Are you currently involved in an exploitative or violent relationship?

□ □ □ Do you radiate intense magnetic or charismatic power, which often attracts many challenging people or situations to you?

Black-Eyed Susan

□ □ □ Do you often find yourself in patterns of denial, blocking things from your memory or disassociating from behavior that you do not really want to face?

□ □ □ Do you suspect a deeply traumatic event from childhood, for which you have "emotional amnesia"?

□ □ □ Is there a shadow side to your personality, or unrecognized part of yourself which needs more honest attention and understanding?

Blackberry

□ □ □ Do you have many plans or intentions which never seem to materialize?

□ □ □ Do you tend to be philosophically oriented, someone more likely to think or reflect than to organize and execute?

□ □ □ Do you feel sluggish, as though your physical body is lacking in essential vitality or willpower?

Bleeding Heart

□ □ □ Do you feel devastated or broken-hearted by a relationship which has ended?

□ □ □ Has a family member or friend recently died, resulting in intense feelings of grief and loneliness?

□ □ □ Do you often find yourself in troubled relationships, especially ones in which you feel rejected?

□ □ □ Do you need a lot of security in personal relationships, or become emotionally dependent on attention from others?

Borage

☐ ☐ ☐ Do you often feel emotionally weighed down, burdened by feelings which seem oppressive or stifling?

☐ ☐ ☐ Are you currently experiencing a great deal of sadness, grief, or loss?

☐ ☐ ☐ Do you feel closed down in your heart, an almost physical sensation of weight or "heavy-heartedness" which prevents you from fully experiencing joy?

Buttercup

☐ ☐ ☐ Do you often find yourself apologizing for what you do or who you are?

☐ ☐ ☐ Do you feel that others are more worthy of attention or respect than you?

☐ ☐ ☐ Do you evaluate your social status by conventional standards of achievement, rather than an inner sense of your own self-worth?

Calendula

☐ ☐ ☐ Do you find yourself frequently interrupting others or becoming argumentative?

☐ ☐ ☐ Is it hard for you to listen or to take genuine interest in what others are saying?

☐ ☐ ☐ Do you feel you need to develop more warmth and compassion in the way you relate to others?

California Pitcher Plant

☐ ☐ ☐ Do you often feel disgusted or squeamish around anything that is too raw or "gut-level"?

☐ ☐ ☐ Do you keep yourself under strict control, so that you are seldom spontaneous or instinctive in your response?

☐ ☐ ☐ Do you tend to be anemic, pale, or lacking in physical vigor or strength?

California Poppy

☐ ☐ ☐ Do you often find yourself fascinated by glamorous or charismatic people, or attracted to experiences which seem to promise more than they actually deliver?

☐ ☐ ☐ Do you use drugs or seek similar experiences which help you to feel "high," or escape the realities of life?

☐ ☐ ☐ Are you a perennial seeker, always looking for someone or some teaching which will hold the real answer?

A	S	N	## California Wild Rose
☐	☐	☐	Is it hard for you to get involved in committed relationships or in community service?
☐	☐	☐	Do you frequently feel apathetic or bored, lacking enthusiasm o interest in life?
☐	☐	☐	Do you often find yourself unwilling to take risks, hoping to avoid the possible pain or challenge involved?

Calla Lily

A	S	N	
☐	☐	☐	Are you deeply troubled or uncomfortable with your sexual iden tity or gender?
☐	☐	☐	Did you receive mixed messages about your sexual identity o gender when you were a child or adolescent?
☐	☐	☐	Do you feel you need to integrate the inner qualities of mascu line and feminine within yourself into a more harmonious wholeness?

Canyon Dudleya

A	S	N	
☐	☐	☐	Does your life often seem like one big trauma-drama, as though you are in continual crisis?
☐	☐	☐	Do you find yourself exaggerating events, somehow needing to have things appear larger than ordinary life?
☐	☐	☐	Do you have hysterical or dramatic tendencies which interrupt the flow of daily life for yourself and those around you?

Cayenne

A	S	N	
☐	☐	☐	Are you currently in a situation which feels "stuck" or stagnant?
☐	☐	☐	Would you like to make some changes in your life, but lack the energy or fire to do so?
☐	☐	☐	Do you find that you have a phlegmatic or complacent personali ty, one which tends to watch life go by?

Centaury

A	S	N	
☐	☐	☐	Are you someone who finds it easy to serve others, but submerges your own identity or integrity in the process?
☐	☐	☐	Is it difficult for you to be in touch with your own needs for rest, play or creative expression; and do you find that you all too easily compromise these needs to meet the demands of others?
☐	☐	☐	Do you feel that your will is weak, especially with regard to your own personal goals for inner development or self-realization?

A   S   N

Cerato

☐ ☐ ☐ Do you doubt your own intuitive assessment of people or situations, frequently relying on the counsel of others?

☐ ☐ ☐ Do you commonly find yourself regretting choices you have made, realizing you were not in touch with your own inner wisdom at the time of the decision?

☐ ☐ ☐ Are you currently required to make life choices or critical decisions which require your utmost ability to form independent judgment and your own authentic evaluation?

Chamomile

☐ ☐ ☐ Do you frequently burst into tears or react in a highly emotional way to many life situations?

☐ ☐ ☐ Do you often feel a lot of tension or congestion in your stomach or solar plexus, as though there are many feelings stored there?

☐ ☐ ☐ Do you believe that you need to develop more serenity in life; that you are often fluctuating between one emotional mood or another?

Chaparral

☐ ☐ ☐ Do you frequently have troubling dreams or nightmares?

☐ ☐ ☐ Do you feel there are violent, disturbing or fearful episodes from your past which may still have a psychic grip on you?

☐ ☐ ☐ Have you used psychoactive or psychiatric drugs which altered your consciousness or behavior, and which feel toxic or invasive to your well-being?

Cherry Plum

☐ ☐ ☐ Is your current life characterized by a great deal of pressure or stress, resulting in enormous feelings of emotional or physical tension?

☐ ☐ ☐ Do you tend to cope with stressful or challenging situations by holding on all the tighter, as though letting go would mean that you had lost control?

☐ ☐ ☐ Have you experienced moments of temporary insanity, or suicidal or destructive impulses, which make it hard for you to trust surrendering to your own natural impulses or inner sense of spirituality?

A S N   # Chestnut Bud

☐ ☐ ☐ Does it feel that you are somehow stymied or stuck, unable t make progress, repeating the same mistakes again and again i relationships and other life situations?

☐ ☐ ☐ Is it hard for you to step aside and observe your life, so that yc can understand and learn from your experiences?

☐ ☐ ☐ Does it seem that you are a slow learner, needing to develo more ability to observe and discriminate in the life situatior which you encounter?

Chicory

☐ ☐ ☐ Do you often experience feelings of frustration, suspecting tha others do not really appreciate your efforts?

☐ ☐ ☐ Do you find yourself wanting attention from others, especiall the desire to have others acknowledge how much you are givin or doing for them?

☐ ☐ ☐ Are you possessive in relationships, wanting others to recogniz how important you are in their lives?

☐ ☐ ☐ Do you find that many of your actions provoke the negativ attention of others?

Chrysanthemum

☐ ☐ ☐ Does the idea of aging really scare you, especially the fact c physical death?

☐ ☐ ☐ Are you in mid-life, or in a stage of transition, requiring you t assess your deepest life goals, values and purpose?

☐ ☐ ☐ Are you currently experiencing a life-threatening illness or othe crisis which prompts you to consider the meaning and purpos of your life and spiritual identify?

Clematis

☐ ☐ ☐ Are you someone who lives more readily and comfortably i your own inner world, rather than in an outer world of dail affairs and responsibilities?

☐ ☐ ☐ Do you have a highly developed imagination or psychic life, bu find it difficult to focus or concentrate in the classroom or worl place?

☐ ☐ ☐ Are you attracted to drugs or other psychic experiences whicl give you a sense of expansiveness, and ease your feeling o constriction in the physical body or physical world?

A   S   N   # Corn

☐ ☐ ☐ Are you extremely uncomfortable if anyone intrudes or impinges on your living space or personal environment?

☐ ☐ ☐ Do you find it especially difficult to be in crowds of people or in urban situations, as though you are out of touch with yourself?

☐ ☐ ☐ Do you often sense that your feet are not quite on the earth, as though you are not adequately anchored in your physical body?

Cosmos

☐ ☐ ☐ Do you often find yourself frustrated when you want to speak, having much more to say than what actually comes out?

☐ ☐ ☐ Is it difficult to bring order, coherency, or fluency to your thinking, speaking, or writing?

☐ ☐ ☐ Do you often feel flooded with inspiration, but at a total loss about how to communicate it to others?

Crab Apple

☐ ☐ ☐ Are you often obsessed with feelings of imperfection, focusing on even the tiniest details which seem out of harmony?

☐ ☐ ☐ Do you feel unclean, impure, or otherwise ashamed of your bodily functions or physical attributes?

☐ ☐ ☐ Are you often drawn to purification or cleansing rituals for your physical body or environment, perhaps out of proportion to the real need?

Dandelion

☐ ☐ ☐ Do you frequently over-schedule yourself, trying to cram as much as you can into every day and every hour?

☐ ☐ ☐ Do you typically experience tension throughout your body, especially in the neck and shoulders?

☐ ☐ ☐ Do you feel the need to flow more with life, especially to give your body a chance to unwind?

Deerbrush

☐ ☐ ☐ Do you often find yourself saying and doing things expected of you, rather than expressing or behaving how you really feel?

☐ ☐ ☐ Are you troubled by your motives, as though there is a dissonance between your outer actions and inner intentions?

☐ ☐ ☐ Do you need more inner awareness, especially to recognize and honor the real feelings in your heart?

A S N   # Dill

□ □ □ Are you frequently in chaotic or stressful environments where it seems that your nerves are stretched to the breaking point?

□ □ □ Are you often bombarded by sights, sounds, and smells which seem to strain your ability to really appreciate or absorb what you encounter?

□ □ □ Do you have plans for (or have you just completed) a major trip, which will require you to encounter many new people, places, and environmental stimuli?

□ □ □ Do you often feel exhausted by the end of the day, as though you've taken in far more than you can inwardly understand or "assimilate"?

Dogwood

□ □ □ Would you describe yourself as accident-prone — someone who seems to have more than your share of accidents, both big and little?

□ □ □ Did you feel extremely insecure as a child, or were there harsh circumstances which left you feeling unprotected, abused, or neglected?

□ □ □ Does your body often feel awkward or heavy to you, as though you would like to feel more grace and ease?

Easter Lily

□ □ □ Do you feel conflict about how to express your sexuality, vacillating between prudishness or promiscuity?

□ □ □ Does it seem hard for you to establish your own standards of integrity, given society's conflicting messages about sexuality?

□ □ □ Is there a current issue for you regarding the purification of your sexual desires, or a sense of dysfunction or disturbance in your sexual and reproductive organs?

Echinacea

□ □ □ Are you currently experiencing a great deal of stress or upheaval in your life, requiring you to rally all the inner strength and positive identity you can muster?

□ □ □ Do you feel somehow numb or devoid of true identity, as though life is so painful it's hard to be really present for it?

□ □ □ Have you experienced a situation which was so abusive or assaulting that you feel robbed of your essential dignity or self-respect, either recently or in the past?

A   S   N   # Elm

☐ ☐ ☐ Do you readily assume major tasks or responsibilities, only to find yourself completely overwhelmed or otherwise dysfunctional?

☐ ☐ ☐ Are you someone who is frequently overly-responsible or over-concerned in family or work situations, to the point of isolating yourself as the lone hero or rescuer?

☐ ☐ ☐ Are you currently experiencing a great deal of fatigue, or even despondency, regarding a task or project for which you have assumed responsibility?

Evening Primrose

☐ ☐ ☐ Do you often feel unwanted or unloved, tracing these feelings back to your earliest childhood memories?

☐ ☐ ☐ Do you frequently feel emotionally cold or distant in relationships, as though it's hard for you to feel love from others or to express it in return?

☐ ☐ ☐ Were you an adopted child, or did your mother have a great deal of conflict or stress while pregnant with you?

Fairy Lantern

☐ ☐ ☐ Were you the youngest child in your family, or did family circumstances excessively reinforce your identity as a child or dependent?

☐ ☐ ☐ Is it difficult for you to have stable employment or commitment to family responsibilities?

☐ ☐ ☐ Do you frequently daydream about your childhood, or wish to return to some part of your past which seemed more carefree and innocent?

Fawn Lily

☐ ☐ ☐ Are you more comfortable with a spiritual or meditative lifestyle, which requires that you retreat from the normal pace of life?

☐ ☐ ☐ Does the modern technological world seem harsh and invasive to you, as though you would have been happier living in a simpler time?

☐ ☐ ☐ Do you require a great deal of alone or quiet time, making it stressful for you if job or family obligations require too much "outer" time?

A   S   N   # Filaree

□ □ □ Would you describe yourself as a "nit-picker," someone who is often preoccupied with even the smallest details at home or work?

□ □ □ Do you often find yourself wondering where the time goes, becoming entangled in myriad details but failing to accomplish your major goals?

□ □ □ Is it common for you to worry or become hyper-focused toward some event, person or object, often out of proportion to its actual importance?

Forget-Me-Not

□ □ □ Is it hard for you to sustain a memory or an inner relationship with a loved one who has died?

□ □ □ Do you feel abandoned or bereft since the passing of a family member or friend?

□ □ □ Are you seeking a deeper, more soulful and eternal understanding of your relationships with family and friends?

□ □ □ Are you intending to conceive a child, or are you currently pregnant and needing to develop a deeper appreciation for the soul bonds which connect you to this being?

Fuchsia

□ □ □ Do you have a lot of confusing and shifting physical symptoms which seem to be precipitated by emotional experiences?

□ □ □ Do you find yourself reacting with surface emotions to many life events, yet somehow unable to express your deeper, authentic feelings?

□ □ □ Do you feel a need to address some deep-seated feelings of grief, pain, anger or rejection in a way that seems more genuine and honest?

Garlic

□ □ □ Do you often look pale or anemic, or feel drained of life force?

□ □ □ Do you tend to be nervous, easily frightened, or apprehensive; in need of more strength and vitality?

□ □ □ Have you been through a physical illness or other circumstance which left you feeling listless or sapped of energy, as though your immune system is compromised?

A S N

Gentian

☐ ☐ ☐ Are you generally skeptical, often dwelling more on the problem than the solution?

☐ ☐ ☐ Are you often discouraged by setbacks, viewing them as stumbling blocks rather than as learning lessons?

☐ ☐ ☐ Do you easily succumb to doubt or pessimism, finding it hard to tackle any difficulty you experience with renewed forces or a fresh start?

Golden Ear Drops

☐ ☐ ☐ Is it hard for you to recall much about your childhood, perhaps suppressing painful experiences you don't want to remember?

☐ ☐ ☐ Do you find it hard to cry, because you learned a long time ago to hold back your real feelings?

☐ ☐ ☐ Are you often haunted or troubled by memories from childhood, and wish to bring deeper awareness and understanding to your early experiences?

Golden Yarrow

☐ ☐ ☐ Do you often get "performance anxiety" when in front of others?

☐ ☐ ☐ Do you hold back from public roles because you feel too vulnerable, or don't know how to remain confident and centered?

☐ ☐ ☐ Are you an artist or in a similar lifestyle which demands great sensitivity and inner awareness, yet also exposes you to public scrutiny?

Goldenrod

☐ ☐ ☐ Do you frequently find yourself ignoring or compromising your real values or feelings in order to gain social approval or acceptance from others?

☐ ☐ ☐ Are you in a family or other group situation which makes it difficult for you to remain true to your own individual feelings?

☐ ☐ ☐ Do you find that you seldom take time to be alone with yourself, or to get in touch with your deepest needs, goals or visions?

Gorse

☐ ☐ ☐ Does it seem that there is little hope for the challenging condition or situation you are now experiencing?

☐ ☐ ☐ Does your personal world feel dark or menacing, with the feeling that you can expect no improvement or betterment of your situation?

☐ ☐ ☐ Have you lost faith or trust in your inner process of healing or transformation, believing that there is little you can do to improve your condition?

A S N   # Heather

☐ ☐ ☐ Does it seem that you are often absorbed in your life traumas or worries, needing to tell others about them, or wanting attention or consolation from others?

☐ ☐ ☐ Is it challenging for you to be alone or to resolve problems independently, instead requiring a great deal of support from others?

☐ ☐ ☐ Do you feel an intense inner loneliness or sense of insecurity, looking to others to help fill the emptiness you feel inside?

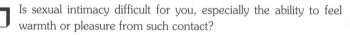

Hibiscus

☐ ☐ ☐ Is sexual intimacy difficult for you, especially the ability to feel warmth or pleasure from such contact?

☐ ☐ ☐ Do you feel that previous sexual trauma or abuse has numbed or disengaged you from a sense of your own true sexual identity?

☐ ☐ ☐ Do you find it difficult to integrate the real warmth and love you feel in your heart with a more physical experience of sexuality?

Holly

☐ ☐ ☐ Are you plagued by feelings of jealously, rivalry, suspicion or vengefulness?

☐ ☐ ☐ Is it hard for you to feel compassion for the plight of others?

☐ ☐ ☐ Do your feelings for others often turn to alienation, mistrust, or hostility?

☐ ☐ ☐ Do you struggle or compete in order to receive love or recognition, feeling that others will get what is rightfully yours?

Honeysuckle

☐ ☐ ☐ Do you find yourself frequently dwelling on, or otherwise longing for a former relationship or living situation?

Does it seem that there was an earlier part of your life which was more glamorous or fulfilling than your current situation?

Do you find yourself wistfully nostalgic or romantic, convinced that life would be different if only you lived in another era, or in a different circumstance?

A	S	N	

Hornbeam

Do you feel fatigued or drained in your job, or in a work-project at home or school, out of proportion to the real physical energy demanded for the task?

Does life often seem like a monotonous routine, as though you are just going through the motions at work or home, with little interest or energetic involvement?

Do you feel you need to develop a fresh perspective on your daily tasks and responsibilities, perhaps recapturing your original zest, or finding new and enlivening situations at work, home, or school?

Hound's Tongue

Do you feel that your scientific or intellectual training has somehow blunted your ability to perceive the world in a more soulful manner?

Is it hard for you to think in an imaginative or lively way; does it seem that your perception is dulled or overly mundane?

Do you tend to see reality as composed of "things" rather than "beings"; as more material than spiritual?

Impatiens

Do you often find yourself tense, irritable, or easily impatient and argumentative?

Do you tend to take over for others, finishing their sentences or completing their tasks because you know you can do it more quickly?

Does it seem that you are always rushing ahead of your experience, not really able to enjoy or pay attention to what is unfolding around you?

Indian Paintbrush

Do you have many artistic ideas or projects which never come to full expression or manifestation?

Do you find any creative process very intense or hard on your body, often leaving you feeling drained and devitalized afterwards?

Do you feel that your creative expressions are too dull or lifeless, needing more earthly vitality?

A S N   # Indian Pink

☐ ☐ ☐   Are you easily attracted to many activities or projects, but often feel that you are spinning out of control?

☐ ☐ ☐   Is it hard for you to remain centered when demands are made on you, as though you lose awareness of your own identity?

☐ ☐ ☐   Are you frequently tense or emotionally volatile, agitated by too much activity and lacking a feeling of calm centeredness?

Iris

☐ ☐ ☐   Is there little art or beauty in your life; does your life seem mundane and strictly practical?

☐ ☐ ☐   Were you told as a child that you weren't an artist, or were your artistic aspirations somehow blunted?

☐ ☐ ☐   Does your emotional life, home or work environment seem dull or gray; do you need to bring more inspiration and soul color into your life?

Lady's Slipper

☐ ☐ ☐   Does it seem that your current life is only a dim reflection of what you are really capable of achieving?

☐ ☐ ☐   Do you often feel exhausted or weary, as though you are out of touch with your own sense of personal power and destiny?

☐ ☐ ☐   Does it seem that you need to integrate your sense of spiritual purpose and vision more closely with your daily work and lifestyle?

Larch

☐ ☐ ☐   Are you your own worst critic, censoring, down-playing, or otherwise stifling your creative expression or contribution?

☐ ☐ ☐   Do you suffer from self-doubt, often lacking the essential confidence to take risks or be spontaneous?

☐ ☐ ☐   Does your own fear of failure or expectation of criticism from others hold you back from making a unique or creative contribution in your work, community or social group?

☐ ☐ ☐   Do you experience difficulty in speaking or performing publicly, adversely affecting your speech or presentation, even when you are sufficiently prepared?

A	S	N	

Larkspur

☐ ☐ ☐ Do you have conflicting feelings about leadership or service, wanting to be in charge, but then shirking your responsibilities?

☐ ☐ ☐ Do you find yourself going through life dutifully executing your responsibilities, rather than being carried along by inner joy and purpose?

☐ ☐ ☐ Do you find that others respond negatively or apathetically to you when you're in a leadership position?

Lavender

☐ ☐ ☐ Would you characterize yourself as "high-strung" — often being hyperactive or nervous?

☐ ☐ ☐ Do you suffer from insomnia, mental tension, or headaches when you are highly concerned or overly absorbed in something?

☐ ☐ ☐ Are you attracted to a very spiritual lifestyle, which includes many hours of meditation or other spiritual practice?

Lotus

☐ ☐ ☐ Is it hard for you to think of yourself as a spiritual person, or to open yourself to spiritual experiences?

☐ ☐ ☐ Do you have a great deal invested in your spiritual identity, so much so that you would not want others to see you as having lower emotions or passions?

☐ ☐ ☐ Do you feel that your spirituality is unbalanced, that it is either expressed too little, or too exaggerated and not integrated enough with daily life?

Love-Lies-Bleeding

☐ ☐ ☐ Are you currently suffering from a physical disease or from some form of mental agony which makes you feel abandoned or isolated?

☐ ☐ ☐ Is it hard for you to reach out to others when you are in pain; do you prefer to be left alone or believe that others will not understand you?

☐ ☐ ☐ Do you feel deeply depressed about a physical handicap, illness, or other form of anguish, which makes it hard for you to see any meaning or purpose in your suffering?

Madia

☐ ☐ ☐ Do you get easily distracted, finding it challenging to stay focused on any one idea or project?

☐ ☐ ☐ Do you tend to start projects or tasks, and then lose interest or leave them unfinished?

☐ ☐ ☐ Do you have trouble with mental concentration, feeling drowsy or listless, especially in the afternoon or in hot weather?

Mallow

☐ ☐ ☐ Do you have a difficult time making friends, finding it hard to feel affectionate or socially outgoing?

☐ ☐ ☐ Are you frustrated by inner feelings of warmth or closeness that are not conveyed easily to those you love?

☐ ☐ ☐ Would you like to develop more trust and openness in your relationships with others?

Manzanita

☐ ☐ ☐ Do you have a negative self-image of your body or physical presence in life?

☐ ☐ ☐ Do you frequently diet or binge, or subject yourself to harsh physical regimens of exercise?

☐ ☐ ☐ Does it often seem like the spiritual and physical parts of you are at war; that your body does not seem harmonious with your spiritual identity?

Mariposa Lily

☐ ☐ ☐ Was your relationship with your mother — or any other major female figure — full of turmoil or alienation?

☐ ☐ ☐ Were you abandoned, abused, or did you suffer any other major trauma during your childhood years?

☐ ☐ ☐ Do you need to develop an understanding of your early childhood experiences, especially your relationship with your mother and how it affects your current life?

☐ ☐ ☐ *For women:* Do you feel a lot of conflict, doubt or insecurity about your own role as a mother?

A S N   Milkweed

☐ ☐ ☐ Have you suffered a long illness, trauma or other handicap which has made you extremely dependent on others?

☐ ☐ ☐ Is it hard for you to feel responsible or truly independent; do you frequently find yourself needing to be cared for by others?

☐ ☐ ☐ Have you used drugs or other extreme behaviors to blot out your conscious awareness or autonomy?

Mimulus

☐ ☐ ☐ Do you find that you frequently shortchange yourself from a full experience of life, isolating yourself due to nagging fears or worries?

☐ ☐ ☐ It is hard for you to be truly spontaneous or joyfully curious about life, paralyzed instead by annoying doubts, fears or worries?

☐ ☐ ☐ Would you describe yourself as hypersensitive, frequently troubled or uneasy even when encountering ordinary or daily activities?

Morning Glory

☐ ☐ ☐ Are your basic living patterns erratic or chaotic — tending to eat, sleep, work or travel at divergent or unpredictable times?

☐ ☐ ☐ Does it seem as though your internal body clock is askew, finding it hard to arise freshly in the morning but staying up late at night?

☐ ☐ ☐ Are you attracted to stimulant foods or drugs which boost your energy level, or give you a false sense of energy your body does not have?

Mountain Pennyroyal

☐ ☐ ☐ Have you recently been subjected to hostile or otherwise negative behavior from others which seems to be affecting how you feel and think?

☐ ☐ ☐ Do your thoughts or feelings seem hazy or troubled, or do you often feel drained and unnecessarily fatigued?

☐ ☐ ☐ When you examine your actions, does it feel as though you're not really in the driver's seat, but rather that you are carrying out the intentions or desires of others?

A S N   # Mountain Pride

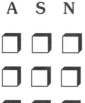

Do you often avoid letting others know what you really think, remaining uncomfortably passive or silent?

Are you currently in a challenging situation which demands that you take a stand, or make a choice for your beliefs?

Do you need to develop more confidence in yourself, especially your ability to be strong, courageous or positively assertive?

Mugwort

Does it often seem as though your inner life of dreams or thoughts is blurred or confused with outer, ordinary events?

Is there a strong intuitive or psychic aspect to your personality, so much so that it sometimes overpowers your good judgment or observation in the physical world?

Do you need to develop greater clarity of consciousness, especially regarding dreams or other inner events and their relationship to your daily life and responsibilities?

Mullein

Do you frequently find yourself lying to others, or acting in other ways which are deceitful or misleading?

Are you currently facing a painful decision which requires that you further develop your sense of inner conscience or moral values?

Do you need to develop more personal authenticity, so that your values or the meaning of your actions are really clear to others?

Mustard

Are you often subject to unexpected bouts of depression or inner darkness?

Does it seem that you readily experience mood swings, at times happy or joyful, then suddenly filled with feelings of gloom or melancholy?

Is it difficult for you to grasp the causes of your depression or anxiety, as though it comes from outside you like a dark cloud?

Nasturtium

Does your current occupation or lifestyle demand a great deal of study or other mental concentration?

Does your approach to life seem at times to be too dry, abstract, or intellectual?

Do you find that you are lacking in fire, vitality or warmth, frequently experiencing colds, congestion or other physical depletion?

A	S	N	

Nicotiana

☐ ☐ ☐ Do you have a disposition that could be described as "macho": a tough, cool persona which seems impervious to emotions?

☐ ☐ ☐ Do you use drugs, especially tobacco, as a way to feel more relaxed, grounded and emotionally stable?

☐ ☐ ☐ Do you often find yourself needing to blunt or numb your feelings, in order to cope with the harsh or stressful environment around you?

Oak

☐ ☐ ☐ Are you hard-working and dependable, often pressing to the limits of endurance in order to provide for or assist others?

☐ ☐ ☐ Do you feel you are on the verge of collapse or utter exhaustion due to the unrelenting pace you have set for yourself?

☐ ☐ ☐ Do you over-strive beyond your true limits or capacities, generally denying yourself small pleasures or spontaneous moments of joy?

Olive

☐ ☐ ☐ Are you facing now, or have you just completed an extremely challenging ordeal which requires you to muster all your physical stamina and resolve?

☐ ☐ ☐ Do you feel that you have "spent" all of your physical energy, resulting in a profound sense of exhaustion and fatigue?

☐ ☐ ☐ Do you generally seek physical measures to heal yourself, yet sense that your current exhaustion or dysfunction is so immense you must look elsewhere for complete recovery?

Oregon Grape

☐ ☐ ☐ Are you often filled with feelings of paranoia or mistrust regarding the intentions of others?

☐ ☐ ☐ During childhood, did you experience the world as an unsafe place, or that you had to constantly defend yourself in order to survive?

☐ ☐ ☐ When you meet others, is your first instinct to wonder how they might harm you, rather than how you might help them?

A   S   N   # Penstemon

☐ ☐ ☐ Have you experienced one or more misfortunes or life tragedies, which require you to rally all the faith and endurance you can possibly muster?

☐ ☐ ☐ Do you suffer a physical defect or other handicap which requires enormous fortitude and strength in order to cope from day to day?

☐ ☐ ☐ Do you have the feeling of being persecuted or otherwise victimized, making it hard for you to sustain faith or trust in the unfolding of your life?

Peppermint

☐ ☐ ☐ Are you often hungry and in need of stimulation from food, only to find yourself dull and mentally sluggish after you've eaten?

☐ ☐ ☐ Do you drink coffee or take other stimulants in order to feel mentally alert enough to accomplish your tasks?

☐ ☐ ☐ Does your mind often feel foggy or lethargic, lacking in alert and awake mental forces?

Pine

☐ ☐ ☐ Did you grow up in a religious, social, or family situation which imparted a great deal of guilt or shame about your own self-worth?

☐ ☐ ☐ Do you have unusually harsh expectations for yourself, readily resorting to self-blame if your performance is less than perfect?

☐ ☐ ☐ Is it hard for you to let go of past mistakes or failures, frequently dwelling on these rather than moving forward to new opportunities or risks?

Pink Monkeyflower

☐ ☐ ☐ Do you suffer from intense feelings of shame or vulnerability, feeling you need to protect yourself from exposure to others?

☐ ☐ ☐ Were you deeply wounded or violated in the past, so much so that it's hard for you to take emotional risks with others?

☐ ☐ ☐ Is it hard for others to touch the deepest feelings in your heart, as though you feel wary or even fearful of their intentions?

Pink Yarrow

☐ ☐ ☐ Are you easily influenced by others' emotions, making it difficult for you to distinguish your own feelings from those of others?

☐ ☐ ☐ Are you often in a caretaking or nurturing role, yet find yourself drained and depleted by the emotional needs of others?

☐ ☐ ☐ Are you hypersensitive to any emotional discord in your environment, making you feel extremely uneasy or otherwise dysfunctional?

A S N

Poison Oak

☐ ☐ ☐ Do you frequently find yourself creating negative barriers to others, especially through anger, hostility or irritability?

☐ ☐ ☐ Do you often keep a "safe" emotional distance, so that you do not have to show too much intimacy, emotion or vulnerability?

☐ ☐ ☐ Do you have a fear of being engulfed or absorbed by others, especially anyone who seems too feminine or nurturing?

Pomegranate

☐ ☐ ☐ *For women:* Are you currently experiencing great doubt or conflict in choosing between having a family or developing your career?

☐ ☐ ☐ *For women:* Are you infertile, or have you recently experienced a miscarriage or abortion, causing you to reconsider or resolve your feelings about pregnancy and motherhood?

☐ ☐ ☐ Are you ambivalent or confused about how to focus your creativity, especially between values of career and home, or personal and social involvement?

Pretty Face

☐ ☐ ☐ Do you invest a great deal of time or money in your personal appearance?

☐ ☐ ☐ Do you feel a sense of shame or unease if your personal appearance or physical body is less than perfect?

☐ ☐ ☐ Do you have a physical handicap, or a condition due to aging or physical disease, which makes it hard to accept yourself as you are?

Purple Monkeyflower

☐ ☐ ☐ Are many of your spiritual feelings fear-based, such as a fear of retribution by your religious community or punishment from God?

☐ ☐ ☐ Would you like to develop a more authentic expression of your own spirituality, but fear censure or condemnation by others?

☐ ☐ ☐ Have you experienced a premature psychic opening through drugs, cultic abuse or other psychic means, which makes you fearful or uncertain of how to practice your spirituality?

A S N

Quaking Grass

☐ ☐ ☐ Do you find it challenging to be involved with groups, tending to be protective of your individual identity?

☐ ☐ ☐ Are you experiencing a lot of conflict about a current social situation, either within your family, workplace or larger community?

☐ ☐ ☐ Do you tend to avoid any kind of group process, finding it irritating, tiresome or frustrating?

Queen Anne's Lace

☐ ☐ ☐ Do you often experience blurred, foggy or distorted vision, especially when you are under emotional stress or psychic overwhelm?

☐ ☐ ☐ Is it easy for you to distort or misunderstand your perception of people or events, as though your "emotional vision" is clouded?

☐ ☐ ☐ Do your psychic and sexual energies often interfere with each other, requiring more inner clarity and balance?

☐ ☐ ☐ Do you have clairvoyant or psychic impressions which seem distorted or emotionally based, needing keener perception and objective insight?

Quince

☐ ☐ ☐ Are you a single parent, or in a similar caretaking role which demands equal measures of strength and sensitivity?

☐ ☐ ☐ Do you find yourself being too harsh with children or others in your care, not sure how to combine discipline with nurturing?

☐ ☐ ☐ Do you find it hard to trust, or to act from the softer side of your personality, fearing that others will lose respect for you?

Rabbitbrush

☐ ☐ ☐ Does your job or home role require the command of lots of details which need to be handled simultaneously?

☐ ☐ ☐ Is it difficult for you to maintain awareness of the "big picture" when you are working on a project that includes many fine points?

☐ ☐ ☐ Does your life often feel overwhelming or chaotic because you are simply not able to keep pace with all the "loose ends" for which you are responsible?

Red Chestnut

☐ ☐ ☐ Do you frequently find yourself worrying or concerned about others' welfare, so much so that you are living more in their lives than your own?

☐ ☐ ☐ Is it hard for you to trust in the unfolding of life events for your children or other family or friends close to you?

☐ ☐ ☐ Are you needing to develop more detachment about a current relationship or social situation which is troubling you?

Red Clover

☐ ☐ ☐ Do you find yourself unable to cope in emergencies, often succumbing to panic or hysteria?

☐ ☐ ☐ Have you found yourself unduly influenced by a public personality or political ideology, responding with fear to a picture of doom or disaster?

☐ ☐ ☐ Do you lose your positive identity in your family or other close group, whenever there are challenging or negative circumstances?

Rock Rose

☐ ☐ ☐ Do you frequently suffer from nightmares, or other experiences which bring a sense of terror or deep emotional disturbance?

☐ ☐ ☐ Are you currently facing a situation which has life-threatening or destructive proportions, such as an impending death or catastrophic emergency?

☐ ☐ ☐ Do you need to develop greater courage and equanimity in stressful situations?

Rock Water

☐ ☐ ☐ Do you tend toward an ascetic or highly regimented style of living and eating?

☐ ☐ ☐ Do you have strong religious, work, or study disciplines, which you follow relentlessly, or rigidly?

☐ ☐ ☐ Do you feel that you deny yourself the opportunity to enjoy life on its own terms, generally subjecting yourself to strict schedules or external programs which allow for little spontaneity or creativity?

A   S   N   # Rosemary

☐ ☐ ☐ Do you frequently experience states of absentmindedness or forgetfulness, as though your consciousness is not fully present at times?

☐ ☐ ☐ Do you tend to have cold extremities — especially hands and feet — with the feeling that it's difficult to bring your consciousness and warmth completely into your physical body?

☐ ☐ ☐ Did you experience trauma sometime in your past, in which extreme physical abuse or stress kept you from feeling warm and secure in your physical body?

Sage

☐ ☐ ☐ Do you need to develop more objectivity and perspective about recent life events which trouble or perplex you?

☐ ☐ ☐ Does your life seem more accidental than purposeful, making it hard to have much insight into, or acceptance of, the people and events surrounding you?

☐ ☐ ☐ Are you in an elder phase of life, wanting to gather wisdom and reflect on the meaning of your experience?

Sagebrush

☐ ☐ ☐ Does your life seem unnecessarily cluttered, burdened or complex, as though you need to learn how to let go and find more simplicity?

☐ ☐ ☐ Have you recently experienced an illness or misfortune, which is prompting you to change and to let go of old parts of your self or lifestyle?

☐ ☐ ☐ Is it difficult for you to contact your true spiritual identity, because you hold on too tightly to possessions, lifestyle, or social personality?

Saguaro

☐ ☐ ☐ Do you feel alienated from or ashamed of your family lineage, cultural or ethnic identity?

☐ ☐ ☐ Do you frequently find yourself rebelling against or in conflict with persons who have authority or power over you?

☐ ☐ ☐ Do you need to develop a deeper understanding or respect for the traditions which have shaped your family or cultural identity?

Saint John's Wort

☐ ☐ ☐ Are you hypersensitive to bright light or heat, feeling particularly drained or dysfunctional during the summer?

☐ ☐ ☐ Do you feel depressed in the winter when there's not enough light?

☐ ☐ ☐ Is it common for you to experience distress when sleeping, such as dream disturbances, night-sweats or bed-wetting?

☐ ☐ ☐ Is your state of consciousness generally diffuse or expansive, needing more inner strength and clarity?

Scarlet Monkeyflower

☐ ☐ ☐ Do you have a difficult time dealing with issues of anger or power, tending instead to "stuff" your feelings?

☐ ☐ ☐ Are you frequently in situations where you try hard to be polite or calm, but suddenly vent explosive feelings of anger or rage?

☐ ☐ ☐ Do you need to develop more direct and clear ways of communication, so that your honest feelings or disagreements are fully acknowledged?

Scleranthus

☐ ☐ ☐ Do you frequently find yourself in situations where you seem torn between one or more options, unable to take a firm hold of your decision?

☐ ☐ ☐ Are you someone who often goes back and forth between people or situations, vacillating in your commitment or intentions?

☐ ☐ ☐ Do you experience a constant shifting of emotional states as well as physical symptoms, characterized by a great deal of restlessness or confusion?

Scotch Broom

☐ ☐ ☐ Do you often get depressed, alienated or overwhelmed when you hear news reports or consider the state of world affairs?

☐ ☐ ☐ Is it hard for you to see how your contribution can make much difference in your neighborhood, community, or in the larger world?

☐ ☐ ☐ Do you frequently experience personal despair, or feel "What's the use, why try?" when it comes to solving problems or helping others?

Self-Heal

☐ ☐ ☐ Do you endlessly try one healing approach after another, convinced that a particular practitioner or health regimen holds the answer for you?

☐ ☐ ☐ Are you currently experiencing a challenging health problem or other dysfunction which requires that you rally all your healing forces?

☐ ☐ ☐ Do you find it hard to see how anything you think, feel or do could make any real difference in your state of wellness?

Shasta Daisy

☐ ☐ ☐ Do you have a challenging time when writing or performing other intellectual tasks, because it's difficult for you to see the main idea or make clear sense of what you are doing?

☐ ☐ ☐ Are you someone who tends to be overly analytical, easily seeing all the bits and pieces but not always grasping or appreciating the larger picture?

☐ ☐ ☐ Does it seems as though your life is full of chaos or divergent threads, requiring you to find more meaning, integration or harmony?

Shooting Star

☐ ☐ ☐ Was there considerable trauma surrounding your birth, or the earliest months of your life?

☐ ☐ ☐ Are you particularly fascinated by stories of UFO's or extra-terrestrial encounters, or do you feel that you've had such an encounter?

☐ ☐ ☐ Do you often feel deeply alienated, as though you don't feel quite at home on earth, or part of the human family?

☐ ☐ ☐ Does your consciousness feel more cosmic than human, leading you to feel less interested in earthly life or mundane, worldly affairs?

Snapdragon

☐ ☐ ☐ Do you tend toward verbal abuse or insults, tending to lash out at others suddenly and without much forethought?

 Does it seem as though you have excess energy in your mouth, needing to chew, eat or talk a great deal?

 Do you have a powerful will or libido, but find it challenging to direct your forces in constructive rather than destructive channels?

A   S   N   # Star of Bethlehem

❑ ❑ ❑ Were you subject to a very deep trauma or assault from which you feel you have never regained your original vitality or strength?

❑ ❑ ❑ Does it seem that a deep sense of inner peace and self-containment is lacking in your life, due to stress and other trauma?

❑ ❑ ❑ Have you suffered from a prolonged state of psychic stress which has led you to feel cut off from your Spiritual Self or deepest soul feelings?

Star Thistle

❑ ❑ ❑ Are you extremely conscious of all of your material possessions or personal wealth, feeling it as a form of personal security?

❑ ❑ ❑ Did you grow up in poverty or in an economically or emotionally unstable situation, which made it hard for you to feel materially secure?

❑ ❑ ❑ Do you have a hard time being open or generous, sharing what you have with others, or taking financial risks?

Star Tulip

❑ ❑ ❑ Do you feel that you lack an inner life, and are unable to contact your own spiritual guidance or inner wisdom?

❑ ❑ ❑ Are you in touch with the feminine side of your consciousness, able to listen to others and to be receptive and intuitive?

❑ ❑ ❑ Do you find it difficult to pray or meditate, or recall your dreams?

Sticky Monkeyflower

❑ ❑ ❑ Have you had a number of sexual relationships which mean very little to the deeper feelings within your heart?

❑ ❑ ❑ Do you hold back from expressing yourself as a sexual human being, because it is hard to feel safe in conveying your inner feelings to another?

❑ ❑ ❑ Are you frightened or awed by sexual intimacy, unsure of how to deal with your own vulnerability or feelings of love and warmth?

Sunflower

❑ ❑ ❑ Is your relationship with your father, or any other significant male figures, full of tension or unresolved conflict?

❑ ❑ ❑ Do you often come on strong or seem overbearing to others, even though you know it is just your way of trying to convey confidence?

❑ ❑ ❑ Do you feel uncertain or insecure about your own core identity or sense of individuality?

A   S   N   Sweet Chestnut

☐ ☐ ☐ Do you feel that you have hit "rock bottom," caught in such an extreme state of despair that there appears to be no way out?

☐ ☐ ☐ Do you feel extreme mental anguish or suffering, as though you have reached the breaking point of what you can endure?

☐ ☐ ☐ Are you experiencing a sense of utter aloneness or abandonment, testing your faith that there really is a Higher Power or loving spiritual source for you?

Sweet Pea

☐ ☐ ☐ Did you move a great deal during childhood or throughout life, so much so that it's hard to feel connected or interested in any place that you live?

☐ ☐ ☐ Do you have a hard time calling the neighborhood, community or geographic area where you live truly "home"?

☐ ☐ ☐ Do you feel out of touch with your environmental surroundings, not really feeling rooted or sustained by the land and the people around you?

Tansy

☐ ☐ ☐ Have you been characterized as "lazy" or an "under-achiever," because it seems that you are not really acting on your full potential?

☐ ☐ ☐ Do you tend to procrastinate, or energetically withdraw from participation or commitment as a way of staying contained and coping with pressure from others?

☐ ☐ ☐ Did your childhood include a great deal of chaos, confusion or emotional instability, which caused you to suppress your natural enthusiasm, curiosity, or energetic response to situations?

Tiger Lily

☐ ☐ ☐ Does it seem that you are overly aggressive or competitive, excessively concerned about your own performance?

☐ ☐ ☐ Do you tend to have separatist tendencies, thinking about your own aims and goals, rather than developing cooperative strategies?

☐ ☐ ☐ *For women:* Are you currently experiencing energetic fluctuations due to menopause, especially stronger, more masculine forces which you need to balance and integrate?

A   S   N   ## Trillium

☐ ☐ ☐ Do you frequently find yourself measuring your own or others' worth by standards of financial wealth and personal power?

☐ ☐ ☐ Would you characterize yourself as extremely ambitious, someone who needs a great deal of wealth and personal influence in order to achieve your life goals?

☐ ☐ ☐ Is your consciousness often directed toward survival issues, feeling that if you had more money or economic security your problems would be solved?

Trumpet Vine

☐ ☐ ☐ Do you speak in a flat, monotone, or unexpressive voice?

☐ ☐ ☐ Do you stutter or stammer when you speak, or have other difficulty fully expressing yourself?

☐ ☐ ☐ Do you need to bring more colorful and creative expression to your speech and your general way of presenting yourself?

Vervain

☐ ☐ ☐ Do you believe that the world would be better off if only others heeded your vision and values?

☐ ☐ ☐ Do you possess great feelings of enthusiasm and intensity, so much so that you can tense and push your body beyond its natural energy level?

☐ ☐ ☐ Do you overwhelm others with your convictions, making it difficult for them to freely develop a response or openly explore your point of view?

Vine

☐ ☐ ☐ Do you often demand obedience or allegiance from others, with a strong need to be in control or to direct others?

☐ ☐ ☐ Are you frequently assertive to the point of being aggressive, wanting to be in charge and insure things will be done "your way"?

☐ ☐ ☐ Do you possess such a strong will that it often seems to overpower or overwhelm those around you?

A S N   Violet

☐ ☐ ☐ Do you suffer from a deep sense of shyness or loneliness, wanting to share more of yourself with others but afraid to do so?

☐ ☐ ☐ Do you often feel fragile or uneasy in group situations, as though your sense of self gets lost or submerged?

☐ ☐ ☐ Do you tend to have a great deal of reserve, frequently working alone or silently; so much so that others might perceive you as being aloof?

Walnut

☐ ☐ ☐ Do you tend to be negatively influenced by family ties or social expectations which hold you back from following your own sense of conviction or destiny?

☐ ☐ ☐ Are you attempting to establish a new program of inner development, or change in lifestyle; yet finding yourself succumbing to old habit patterns, thoughts, or beliefs which retard your progress?

☐ ☐ ☐ Are you in a major state of transition — either physical or psychological — which will require you to view yourself and others in an utterly new or courageous way?

Water Violet

☐ ☐ ☐ Does it seem that you are often rather aloof or socially distant making it hard for people to really get to know you?

☐ ☐ ☐ Do you find yourself measuring others according to social status or economic background, often with the sense that you would not want to associate with someone beneath your level?

☐ ☐ ☐ Are you at your best when you work independently, finding that when you work with others you are easily annoyed or otherwise stymied?

White Chestnut

☐ ☐ ☐ Does your mind sometimes seem like an echo chamber, constantly replaying bits of conversations or life episodes without any apparent resolution?

☐ ☐ ☐ Do you suffer from a great deal of mental agitation or racing thoughts, often resulting in insomnia, fitful sleep, or general restlessness?

☐ ☐ ☐ Is it usually difficult for you to pray or meditate, or to experience an inner state of calm objectivity or inner peace?

A S N   # Wild Oat

◻ ◻ ◻ Do you feel that your current vocation or lifestyle is not in keeping with your sense of inner destiny and life purpose?

◻ ◻ ◻ Do you have many talents and capabilities, yet find it difficult to really focus or harness these gifts toward a worldly vocation?

◻ ◻ ◻ Are you chronically dissatisfied with your work or employment, unable to feel real commitment or interest even after trying many different situations?

Wild Rose

◻ ◻ ◻ Has a prolonged illness or other life situation drained you of vitality or enthusiasm for life?

◻ ◻ ◻ Do you frequently feel resigned or apathetic, as though life seems hardly worth the effort it requires?

◻ ◻ ◻ Do you tend to recover from illness or other setbacks very slowly, seemingly unable to harness the full forces of physical vitality which you need for recovery?

Willow

◻ ◻ ◻ Do you tend to hold on to past injustices or misfortunes, leading to feelings of bitterness or resentment?

◻ ◻ ◻ Do you frequently find yourself in the role of "victim," feeling that you are being persecuted or unfairly punished?

◻ ◻ ◻ Are you emotionally inflexible, finding it difficult to forgive others, or to be accepting and yielding?

Yarrow

◻ ◻ ◻ Are you someone who is extremely sensitive and keenly aware of your environment and of the thoughts and intentions of others, even when not spoken?

◻ ◻ ◻ Do you have many allergic responses to food or environmental stimuli, feeling that you need more inner strength and integrity?

◻ ◻ ◻ Do you often find yourself depleted when you are in crowds, while traveling, or in taxing or challenging social situations?

◻ ◻ ◻ Does your work as a healer, teacher or parent require enormous forces of compassion and giving, which often leaves you feeling you have nothing more to give?

A S N # Yarrow Special Formula

☐ ☐ ☐ Do you travel frequently, especially through airports?

☐ ☐ ☐ Do you work often around video display terminals, or other devices transmitting radiation?

☐ ☐ ☐ Have you had numerous X-rays taken, either recently or in the past?

☐ ☐ ☐ Do you live in a geographic area which is polluted or toxic, or with strong electromagnetic frequencies?

Yellow Star Tulip

☐ ☐ ☐ Is it hard for you to make contact with others, to understand what they are really feeling or saying?

☐ ☐ ☐ Do you need to look at some of the consequences of your actions, to understand more fully how you've hurt others even when you may not have been aware of it?

☐ ☐ ☐ Do you need to develop more empathetic sensitivity in your role as a parent, teacher or manager, or in other social interactions?

Yerba Santa

☐ ☐ ☐ Do you sense within yourself a deep, unexplained grief or profound sadness, which has never been fully realized or explored?

☐ ☐ ☐ Do you feel physical constriction in your chest, or suffer from afflictions to the heart and lungs such as asthma, pneumonia, tobacco addiction or breathing disturbances?

☐ ☐ ☐ Do you tend to tighten your breath as a way of coping with painful feelings, or otherwise hold on to deep feelings of sadness, grief or other soul afflictions?

Zinnia

☐ ☐ ☐ Does your life seem overly grim or serious, as though you are gritting your teeth to get through each day?

☐ ☐ ☐ Are you someone who could be described as "over-dutiful" or a "workaholic," carrying a load of somber responsibilities which seem never-ending?

☐ ☐ ☐ Are you able to laugh at yourself, or find moments of spontaneity or humor on a daily basis?

☐ ☐ ☐ Do you frequently take time to play with children, or to schedule activities for yourself which are truly enjoyable and uplifting?